Brice-Cabrel TAMDJUM KAMGA

PREECLAMPSIA IN PREGNANT WOMEN

Brice-Cabrel TAMDJUM KAMGA

PREECLAMPSIA IN PREGNANT WOMEN

Frequency and Factors: Cases of women seen at the MBOUO Protestant Hospital

ScienciaScripts

Imprint

Cover image: www.ingimage.com

This book is a translation from the original published under ISBN 978-620-6-71228-2.

Publisher:
Sciencia Scripts
is a trademark of
Dodo Books Indian Ocean Ltd. and OmniScriptum S.R.L publishing group

120 High Road, East Finchley, London, N2 9ED, United Kingdom
Str. Armeneasca 28/1, office 1, Chisinau MD-2012, Republic of Moldova, Europe
Printed at: see last page
ISBN: 978-620-7-61994-8

CONTENTS

DEDICACES

I dedicate this work to my parents: my late father Kamga Gougo Jean and my mother Kapoko Kamga Julienne.

THANKS

Before developing our subject, we first give thanks to our Lord JESUS CHRIST, who has supported and blessed us throughout our journey.

Thank you to all the people who supported and accompanied me throughout this work and also during my years of study, namely :
My supervisor: Mr Sayouba Jean Pierre; You do me the honour of judging this work, please find here the expression of my sincere thanks and my deep respect. Thank you for sharing your knowledge and experience with me.
My supervisor, Mr Komguem Gustave: I would like to thank you for guiding me through this project. I would like to express my deep gratitude for your help, your patience, your rigour and your availability. Your passionate teaching and your commitment have set an example for me. Please accept my deepest respect and gratitude.
To the Director of the Mbouo private health staff training complex
Mr NGWOUANOU Daniel Martin for his advice and unconditional support.

My teachers: Dr Kuate Kamga Edith, Mr Kemgne Emmanuel, Dr Simo Josué, Mr Ngwos Alain, Mr Mba Fosso, Dr Minyaka and all the others.
My uncle Foko Hermann Gilbert and his wife Foko Carmen for all their sacrifices and advice to me.
My brothers Kengne Kamga Karen, Kamga Emanuel rossignol, Wouafo Choupé Arnauld, Fono Roméo, and my sisters Djepa Wouafo Rosine, Bakam Kamga Augustine who have supported me and always believed in me.

All the laboratory staff at Mbouo Protestant Hospital, including Mr Tamdem Samuel and Ms Medomgue Nadine, to name but a few.
We cannot close this foreword without thanking all our fellow students who, through their encouragement and advice, have been a great support to us

throughout our academic life: Djeukam Emilie, Djouka Sob Charly, Youbi Tchatchoua Yannick, Mougnol William Rodrigue, Tedongmo Tiobou Gaël and all my other fellow students.

Finally, we would like to thank the doctors, nurses and staff of the Mbouo Protestant Hospital for their guidance and help in collecting the data for this study.

SUMMARY

Pre-eclampsia is a maternal pathology specific to pregnancy, secondary to placental dysfunction occurring from the second trimester of pregnancy and specific to human gestation. The causes of this placental dysfunction are highly variable, making the experimental approach to this pathology extremely complex. Placental dysfunction is responsible for the release into the maternal circulation of substances responsible for endothelial dysfunction, characterised by activation of endothelial cells and increased vascular permeability. It appears to be a two-stage disease, with an initial stage of placental syndrome followed by maternal syndrome. The maternal syndrome in pre-eclampsia corresponds to a state of generalised endothelial dysfunction secondary to an excess of circulating factors toxic to the endothelium which are released by the pathological placenta. Understanding the mechanisms leading to placental ischaemia in pre-eclampsia should shed light on the pathogenesis of pre-eclampsia. With a view to contributing to the prevention of pre-eclampsia, we proposed to conduct a retrospective cross-sectional analytical study of 86 pregnant women. The aim was to assess the factors that contribute to pre-eclampsia, to determine the socio-demographic characteristics of our study population, and to determine the frequency of people at risk of pre-eclampsia. Our survey enabled us to identify the risk factors and to record the BP, proteinuria and uric acid levels in these pregnant women. The results obtained were then stored and analysed using EXCEL and SPSS software. The minimum age was 17 and the maximum 43. The average age was 28.28 with a standard deviation of 5.48. The most represented age group was 22-26. 61% were housewives and the rest were women. 59% of our respondents had never heard of pre-eclampsia.51% were married and 72% of our respondents came from rural areas.Risk factors were identified in 48.5% of our study population and the association of hyperuricemia, proteinuria and hypertension was observed in 6.75% of our respondents.Risk factors such as obesity and overweight had a frequency of 35% and 15%.The frequency of other risk factors in our study population was 59.3%. In the light of these results, we can see that education, information and communication at ANC level are being neglected. We therefore need to sound the alarm, in particular by stepping up IEC sessions in our facilities in order to prevent this pathology.

INTRODUCTION

Pre-eclampsia, also known as toxaemia gravidarum, is a renal complication that occurs during pregnancy. It is a condition characterised by a combination of high blood pressure (hypertension), proteinuria, weight gain and oedema.

It is more common in twin pregnancies and first pregnancies. It's a fairly common condition, since according to **INSERM**, it affects around 5% of pregnant women: 40,000 women are therefore affected by it every year. It also has the unfortunate consequence of being the cause of almost a third of very premature births in France. The main cause, which has been identified in recent years, is a malfunction in the vascularisation of the placenta.

It is defined as high blood pressure and hypersecretion of proteins in the urine. Affecting 3% of pregnant women, it can cause kidney, liver and brain complications in the mother, and even stunted growth or prematurity in the baby. If left untreated and properly managed, this disease can cause numerous complications that can lead to the death of the mother and/or child. (Agnès Ditisheim, 2014)

Pre-eclampsia is a worrying condition because of its high prevalence (10-15% of pregnant women). According to **Nores** et **al**, arterial hypertension (AH) during pregnancy is a topical problem whose epidemiological importance is growing, to the point where, according to **the WHO,** 8.10% of these blood pressure disorders during pregnancy constitute a major global health problem. In black Africa, the prevalence of pre-eclampsia is around 25% (the figure varies from 0.93% to 70%), while death from eclampsia occurs in 0.1% to 10% of cases (**Pierrick HORDÉ, 2014**). In Cameroon, the exact epidemiological situation of pre-eclampsia and eclampsia is still poorly known.

ISSUES

Every day, 1,500 women die from complications related to pregnancy or childbirth. In 2005, there were an estimated 536,000 maternal deaths worldwide. Most of these deaths occur in developing countries and could be prevented. Improving maternal health is one of the eight Millennium Development Goals (MDGs) adopted by the international community at the United Nations Millennium Summit. The fifth goal aims to reduce the maternal mortality rate by three quarters between 1990 and 2015. However, between 1990 and 2005, this rate fell by just 5%. In order to achieve this goal, progress will have to be accelerated. 99% of maternal deaths occur in developing countries. More than half of them occur in sub-Saharan Africa, and a third in South Asia. In developing regions, the maternal mortality rate is
450 maternal deaths per 100,000 live births, compared with 9 in developed regions. A total of 14 countries have a rate in excess of 1,000 and, with the exception of Afghanistan, all are in sub-Saharan Africa: Angola, Burundi, Cameroon, Chad, Democratic Republic of Congo, Guinea-Bissau, Liberia, Malawi, Niger, Nigeria, Rwanda, Sierra Leone and Somalia **(WHO, UNICEF, UNFPA and World Bank estimates, 2007**).

Pre-eclampsia is still a public health problem because of its perinatal consequences for both the foetus and the mother: in the mother, it can lead to intracerebral haemorrhage, haematoma, etc. In the foetus, it can also lead to anaemia. which can lead to the mother's death. In the foetus, it leads to growth retardation due to disruption of foeto-placental exchanges and IUGR. (Kaiman, 2014 The criteria for severity need to be known in order to identify patients at very high risk and refer them to the appropriate facilities according to their level of risk and the term of the birth. In the African environment, late diagnosis at the stage of obstetric complications, inadequate therapeutic indications and insufficient resuscitation resources explain the particular seriousness of pre-eclampsia, which is one of the main causes of maternal and perinatal mortality. (Abalos.E, 2009)

RESEARCH QUESTION :

What is the contribution of hypertension, proteinuria and uric acid to the biological diagnosis of pre-eclampsia in pregnant women?

RESEARCH HYPOTHESIS

A combination of high blood pressure, proteinuria and hyperuricemia can lead to a risk of pre-eclampsia

MAIN OBJECTIVE

-Helping to prevent pre-eclampsia in pregnant women

SPECIFIC OBJECTIVE

This will involve :

-assess the factors contributing to pre-eclampsia

- determine the socio-demographic characteristics of our study population

-determine the frequency of people at risk of pre-eclampsia

CHAPTER 1

LITERATURE REVIEW

I- definition

Pre-eclampsia is a common condition during pregnancy. It combines high blood pressure and proteinuria (presence of protein in the urine). Often benign, this condition can, if left untreated and properly managed, cause numerous complications that can lead to the death of the mother and/or child. Classically considered to be a disease of the hypotheses, pre-eclampsia now appears to be the consequence of a maternal endothelial disease linked to the presence of an abnormal placenta. Pregnancy-induced hypertension, oliguria, impaired urinary sodium excretion and hyper-uricaemia are all late events in the development of the physiological process, although they are essential from a clinical point of view. Before proposing an integrated pathophysiological scheme, we will describe the placental abnormalities and placental disorders at the origin of pre-eclampsia. (Agnès Ditisheim, 2014)

II- epidemiology

The 1.4% rate of hypertension found is certainly an underestimate compared with the overall prevalence of pre-eclampsia, which is estimated at between 3 and 5% of pregnancies worldwide, with a much higher incidence in developing countries. In Europe and the United States, the prevalence is estimated to be between 0.7% and 1.5%, depending on the author (and is thought to be falling in these countries compared with the rates recorded some twenty years ago). In black Africa, prevalence is generally poorly assessed; only hospital statistics are available, with rates varying from 2.8% to 6.1% of deliveries(. In France, particularly in the Paris region, two prospective studies using the same definition criteria report a frequency of between 1.1 and 1.5% of pregnancies). In Asia, the rates reported by a World Health Organisation collaborative study range from

1.5% to 8.3% of pregnant women. The incidence is usually highest in patients under the age of 18, although this is a classic finding in the literature. Instead, there is a double-humped distribution with a peak around the age of 25 and a second peak around the age of 35; this distribution is no longer observed in developed countries. Moreover, young age is increasingly being questioned as a determining risk factor. In fact, it simply corresponds to the usual age at the time of the first pregnancy. The role attributed to a certain maternal immune intolerance in the genesis of pre-eclampsia suggests that it is retroplacental haematoma (7.5% of patients and 28% of complications). These two conditions play an important role in obstetric practice, with an incidence of 1,000 per 100,000 births for eclampsia and 2,970 per 100,000 births for retroplacental haematoma. By way of comparison, in developed countries, eclampsia complicates an average of 1 to 5% of pre-eclampsias, i.e. an incidence of 25 to 50 per 100,000 births, while retroplacental haematoma complicates 3 to 5% of pre-eclampsias. As far as HELLP syndrome is concerned, the low incidence encountered in our series (0.6%) contrasts with the severity of the cases managed (88%). It is certainly underestimated, as the literature estimates its frequency at between 4 and 12% of severe pre-eclampsia. Analysis of the risk factors for complications shows that they are more frequently associated with primigravida, the severity of arterial hypertension and the early onset of pre-eclampsia. The perinatal prognosis of pre-eclampsia is also considered to be very poor due to the frequency of death in utero (5 to 10%) and foetal hypotrophy (15 to 20%).

This study was no exception, with perinatal mortality rates of 470 per 1,000 and foetal hypotrophy of 15%. This The excess mortality rate, also noted in previous studies, is mainly linked to the frequency of maternal complications that are highly fœticidal, such as eclampsia and retroplacental haematoma. Analysis of the risk factors for perinatal mortality shows that it is most often associated with prematurity, foetal hypotrophy and the existence of maternal complications.

These risk factors are found in the literature. However, the level of diastolic blood pressure at delivery is not significantly correlated with perinatal mortality, in line with the findings of other authors**. (ducarne, 2009).**

III- Pathophysiology of pre-eclampsia

Pre-eclampsia is a disease of the maternal endothelium, originating in the placenta. The second phase is clinical and corresponds to dysfunction of the maternal endothelium linked to various substances released by the placenta into the maternal circulation (free radicals, oxidised lipids, cytokines, sVEGFR-1, soluble end globulin). The pathology follows a placental defect. The fact that the spiral arteries of the uterine mucosa do not descend low enough leaves these arteries with their muscle cells (vascular walls). They retain their vasoconstriction capacity, which they would normally lose when the placenta is inserted deep into the uterus. This poor vascularisation of the placenta by the spiral arteries causes the placenta to suffer mainly from hypoxia. The placenta reacts by releasing a whole series of substances that are toxic to the maternal body. These substances are initially released to compensate for the lack of vascularisation, leading in particular to arterial hypertension and reduced perfusion of other organs. The interaction between the suffering placenta and the maternal body is different for each mother, and the organs that may fail vary from one person to another. As a result of this lack of perfusion of the The placenta is macroscopically hypotrophic. Histologically, lesions of infarction, villous hypoxia-ischaemia and sometimes even atheroma and chronic villitis can be observed **(Auger .N, 2015).**

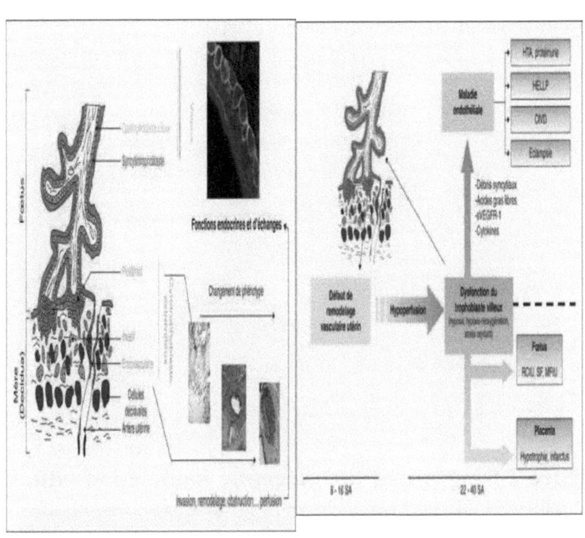

Figure 1: Endocrine function and placental exchange

Physiological reminder

During pregnancy, renal plasma flow and glomerular function increase by 30-50%. Systolic and diastolic blood pressure generally fall by 10 to 15 mmHg compared with pre-pregnancy values. This is due to vasodilatation of the uterine, renal and cutaneous territories, release of vasodilatory prostaglandins by the fetal-placental unit and reduced sensitivity of the arterioles to angiotensin. It plays a role in lowering blood pressure during pregnancy. It is therefore abnormal to have diastolic blood pressure above 85 mmHg in the third trimester. However, an increase in blood pressure during pregnancy is a common and potentially dangerous complication. Blood pressure in excess of 140/90 mmHg is considered pathological **(BENIRSCHKE K, 2008).**

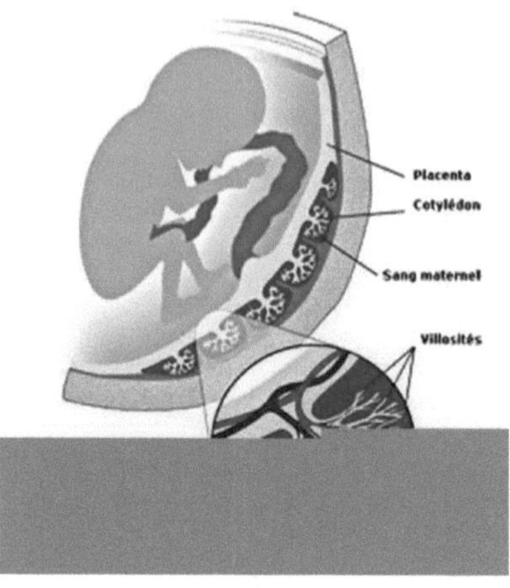

Figure 2 Diagram of the placenta, made up of villi. DR

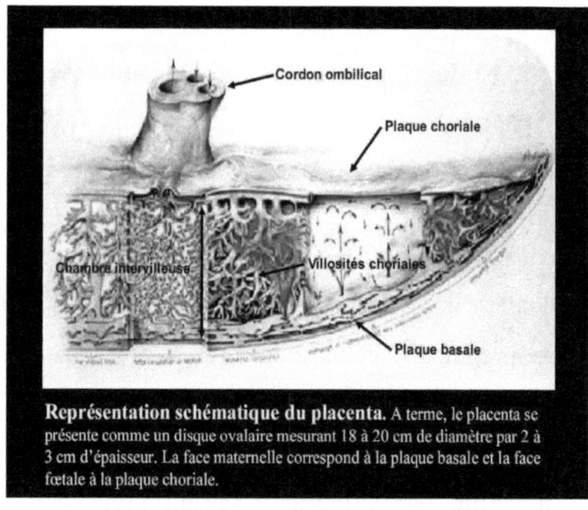

Représentation schématique du placenta. A terme, le placenta se présente comme un disque ovalaire mesurant 18 à 20 cm de diamètre par 2 à 3 cm d'épaisseur. La face maternelle correspond à la plaque basale et la face fœtale à la plaque choriale.

(Y.Fargeaudou, S.Grivaud, 2007)

Figure 3: Schematic cross-section of the placenta A delivery fixed in advance

The diagnosis is made in the presence of high blood pressure, protein in the urine and elevated uric acid in the blood. Various medications may be prescribed (antihypertensive drugs, anticonvulsants, corticosteroids, etc.), and delivery is scheduled by caesarean section. **(Kajantie E, 2009)**

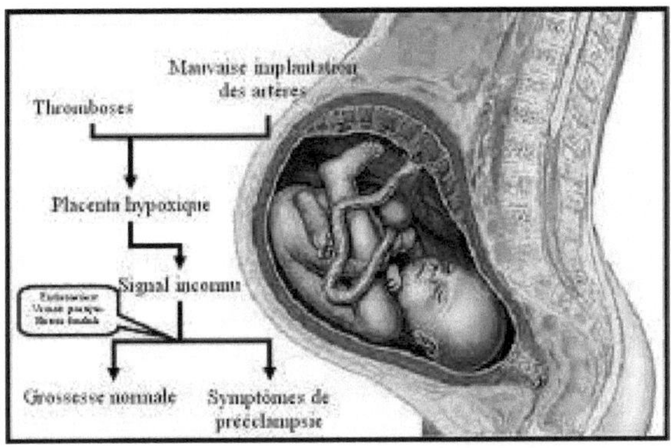

Figure 4: Mechanism leading à a symptom of pre-eclampsia

Scrupulous monitoring

To detect pre-eclampsia as early as possible, the pregnant woman's blood pressure is checked regularly and urine tests are carried out. Aspirin may be prescribed as a preventive measure, under medical supervision, for women already affected during a previous pregnancy.

A rare but sometimes serious pregnancy pathology

Pre-eclampsia is an illness linked to pregnancy (or "gravidarche"), of which it represents a serious complication. It is life-threatening for both mother and foetus. Formerly known as "toxaemia gravidarum", it is caused by a malformation of the blood vessels in the placenta. This pathology is characterised by the presence, in the pregnant woman: **(Kajantie E, 2009)** High blood pressure accompanied by oedema (swelling); loss of protein in the urine. An increase in the level of uric acid in the blood. In addition, as a result of these placental anomalies, the foetus does not receive Pre-eclampsia generally occurs during the second half of pregnancy, from 20 weeks of amenorrhoea (since the last menstrual period). Its name comes from the fact that it can lead to an eclampsia seizure, a serious phenomenon involving convulsions (like an epileptic seizure). Other serious complications may also occur, requiring the patient to be hospitalised until the baby is born. The condition ceases with childbirth and expulsion of the placenta. All the medical treatments used serve to prolong the pregnancy to a term compatible with the survival of the foetus. After the birth of the child, symptoms subside within a few days. **(Kajantie E, 2009)**

Pregnancy-induced arterial hypertension

It is characterised by blood pressure above 14/9, and occurs in women who have never had hypertension before. Like pre-eclampsia, it is caused by a defect in the blood vessels of the placenta. However, it causes little or no loss of protein in the urine. Its presence is therefore not sufficient to diagnose pre-eclampsia. Nevertheless, pregnant women with high blood pressure should be monitored regularly to ensure that their condition does not progress to pre-eclampsia. **(Ness R.B, 2008)**

More or less frequent pathologies

High blood pressure in pregnant women is relatively common, affecting around 10% of pregnancies. Of the women affected, around 10% have pre-existing chronic hypertension. In the others, the onset of the condition is linked to the fact of being pregnant.

In all cases, this condition is likely to lead to pre-eclampsia, which affects around 3% of pregnancies. Eclampsia is rare (less than 1% of pre-eclampsia cases). **(Khan KS. Wojdyla.D Say L et Al, 2006)** Pre-eclampsia and its complications are among the main causes of maternal and foetal death. If the disease appears in a severe form at an early stage (before 26 weeks' amenorrhoea), a medical termination of pregnancy may be recommended to the family.

IV- causes

The causes and mechanisms of pre-eclampsia are not completely understood. We do know, however, that this condition is due to abnormalities in the formation of blood vessels in the placenta, the organ that enables exchanges between the mother and the foetus. The placenta then becomes increasingly "toxic" for both mother and foetus, due to a dangerous increase in blood pressure associated with a high concentration of proteins in the blood. Diet is also one of the most frequent causes. **(Agnès Ditisheim, 2014)**

-Risk factors for pre-eclampsia

The disease is more frequently observed in cases of :

-first pregnancy: little exposure to the father's sperm before becoming pregnant, for example because of a recent change of partner or contraception using a condom (specialists suggest that this could be an immune reaction triggered by exposure to the child's father's antigens);

-a history of pre-eclampsia in the patient or her family (mother, sister)

pre-existing illnesses (obesity, chronic arterial hypertension, chronic kidney disease, anti-phospholipid antibody syndrome, etc.); pregnancy in a woman aged over 40

-a history of caesarean section, death in utero or foetal macrosomia
-multiple pregnancies.

V Acute maternal complications

In addition to eclampsia, pre-eclampsia can give rise to a number of pathologies in pregnant women:

-Retroplacental haematoma: This is a premature detachment of the placenta, causing a haematoma (pocket of blood) between the placenta and the uterus. This painful phenomenon hinders (or even interrupts) blood exchanges between the mother and the foetus. A caesarean section must be performed as a matter of urgency.

-HELLP syndrome (Hemolysis, ElevatedLiver enzymes and LowPlatelets count): This syndrome combines the destruction of red blood cells, liver cells and blood platelets. In this case, a caesarean section must also be performed as soon as possible.

-Other maternal complications: These may include blood clotting in small blood vessels (disseminated intravascular coagulation), acute renal failure, rupture of the uterus, or other complications. haemorrhagic liver disease, stroke, acute lung oedema or retinal detachment **(Agnès Ditisheim, 2014).**

VI- clinical and biological diagnosis A - clinical signs.

A-1 Oedema.

Normally, oedema occurs during pregnancy:

- in the lower limbs, 3 times out of 4.
- in the upper limbs, or generalized in 20 to 25% of cases.

Pathological oedema is oedema that appears suddenly or worsens suddenly. These pathological oedemas modify the weight curve (weight homeostasis axis). They are only a sign of the disease.

A-2 High blood pressure.

The conditions for measuring blood pressure must be strictly adhered to: on the right arm, in a seated position and after at least 10 minutes' rest, with a suitably sized cuff. The minimum is sometimes difficult or impossible to assess by auscultation. Blood pressure should not be taken in the supine position: in this position, postural phenomena can lead to pinching of the blood pressure (hypotensive decubitus syndrome). Normally, pregnancy reduces blood pressure by 10 to 20 MmHg. This relative hypotension appears early, and tends to disappear at the end of pregnancy. During pregnancy, blood pressure retains its nycthemeral rhythm: blood pressure is lower at night. Blood pressure is abnormal when :

- systolic is greater than or equal to 140 MmHg,
- and/or when the diastolic is greater than or equal to 90 MmHg. Similarly, an increase of 30 MmHg in systolic or 15 MmHg in diastolic is considered abnormal (definition now abandoned). In toxaemia, independently of the blood pressure figures, there is a reversal of the nycthemeral rhythm of blood pressure: it is often higher at night. Moreover, especially in severe forms, there is instability: this instability is sometimes 20 to 40 MmHg for the maximum, and 15 to 30 for the minimum. **(Ness R.B, 2008)**

B - Biological signs.

B-1Disturbance of renal function.

Disturbances should be interpreted in the light of the physiological changes induced by pregnancy. Pregnancy is normally accompanied by increases of more than 50% in glomerular filtration, tubular reabsorption and renal blood flow. Thus, normally :

- blood nitrogen levels below 0.20 g/l
- creatinine is less than 10 mg/l (91 µmol/l)

- uricemia is less than 40 mg/l in mid-pregnancy (235 µmol/l)
Less than 55 mg/l at term (324 µmol/l) In practice, uricemia is the most important biological assay. It is sufficient in mild forms. Hyperuricaemia seems to be linked to tubular disturbances. In toxaemia, it correlates well with foetal complications. It is best defined by taking into account variations from values recorded at the start of pregnancy (elevation of 150 µmol/l). If such values are not available, the following limits may be chosen: 250 µmol (40 mg/l) before 32 weeks' gestation, 360 µmol (55 mg/l) after 32 weeks' gestation. Creatinine levels are generally > 80 µmol/l**).** (G.beucher, 2010)

B-2 Proteinuria.

- It can be detected by labstix: if proteinuria is present at 1+, a 24-hour urine test should be carried out. The test cannot be interpreted if the urine pH is alkaline.

- Proteinuria is pathological if it equals or exceeds 0.30 g/24 h. Discreet proteinuria, less than this figure, may be due to an increase in physiological glomerular filtration or contamination of the urine by leucorrhoea.

- Any proteinuria should prompt a search for a urinary tract infection**. (Kajantie E, 2009)**

Pathological examination of the placenta

-A pathology caused by a defect in the placenta

Pre-eclampsia, linked to a malformation of the blood vessels in the placenta, is more common in first-time pregnancies in particular. It can manifest as oedema, headaches or ringing in the ears, moving black or light spots, severe pain just below the ribs, or even an eclampsia attack (convulsions). It is also associated with the following signs:

-hypertension

- proteinuria > 10 mg/dl, sometimes nephrotic;

-oedema.

• We are also pleased to welcome :

- hyperuricemia (>72mg/l) ;

- a generally moderate rise in creatinine levels. (Kaiman, 2014)

VII- Role of uric acid in pre-eclampsia

Recent studies suggest that hyperuricaemia plays a role in the development of hypertension and maternal syndrome. Hyperuricaemia in pre-eclampsia is mainly due to reduced renal excretion as a result of reduced glomerular filtration. There is also probably excessive production of uric acid by the ischaemic placenta. Elevated uricemia often precedes the development of hypertension and proteinuria, and uricemia levels are correlated with a poor prognosis, suggesting that uric acid may have a causal role. Experimental work in rats made hyperuricaemic by the administration of oxonic acid (a uricase inhibitor) shows the appearance of hypertension, glomerular hypertrophy and albuminuria. However, these animals have no endotheliosis, suggesting that uric acid probably plays a contributory but not an initial role in the development of pre-eclampsia. **(schaffer N, 2008)**

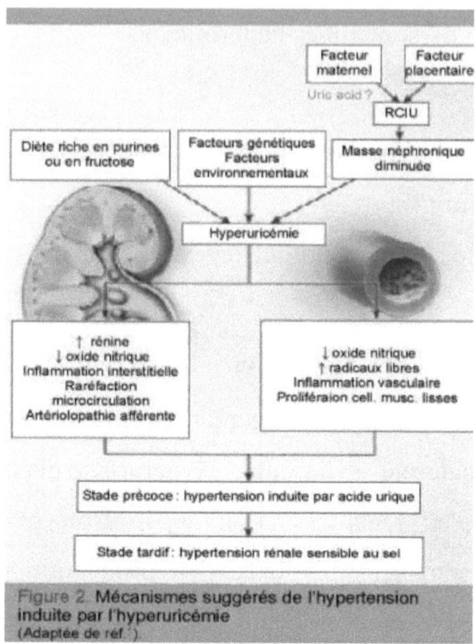

Figure 5: Suggested mechanism of hyperuricemia-induced hypertension

VII- consequences of the disease 1°) Foetal risks.

The impact on the foetus is not correlated with the severity of the maternal pathology.

a- Chronic foetal suffering.

In all vasculo-renal syndromes, the foetus is at risk of chronic foetal suffering and delayed growth, due to disruption of foetal-placental exchanges.

Hence :

- A woman with chronic kidney disease, chronic hypertension or a history of toxaemia should be closely monitored. Additional toxaemia is often serious because the foetal repercussions are severe. By definition, this is referred to as superadded toxaemia:

- if there is an increase of 30 mm in the systolic or 15 mm in the diastolic.

- if proteinuria develops (in cases of chronic arterial hypertension).

- Detection of added toxaemia is aided by biological monitoring of patients at risk: elevation of uric acid, minor coagulation disorders (elevation of VIII R:AG), the appearance of haemoconcentration. Biological changes, in particular elevation of VIII R:AG, may precede maternal clinical signs.

- When toxaemia is suspected, the pregnancy must be monitored very closely. The disease can progress rapidly: in the space of a week, it can go from gestational hypertension to severe toxaemia, or even eclampsia. What's more, in terms of the foetus, chronic foetal distress can rapidly be complicated by sub-acute, then acute foetal distress and foetal death.

- High blood pressure is only one of the signs of the disease. The disease begins before the maternal signs appear. There are many arguments to suggest that the disease may begin around 16-18 weeks' gestation, when the definitive vascular system destined for the placenta is put in place (colonisation of the spiral arteries destined for the placenta by trophoblast). As in all cases of chronic foetal distress, there is a risk of prematurity and IUGR. **(MAYNARD SE, 2006)**

b - Subacute foetal distress.

The disturbance in foetal-maternal exchanges explains the intra-uterine growth retardation. If this disorder worsens, gas exchange may be compromised, and foetal hypoxia and acidosis may develop, with a possible risk of cerebral lesions: this justifies very close monitoring of the foetal state during pregnancy, because acutisation is announced by abnormalities in the FFR or foetal behaviour, or by umbilical doppler abnormalities; by extracting the child in the presence of these abnormalities, we can best preserve its neurological future.

2°) Maternal risks.

- Severe hypertension is life-threatening for the mother. The most common cause of death in eclampsia is intracerebral haemorrhage. The risk is high if PAS > 140 mm Hg emergency parenteral treatment

- In addition, there are two progressive complications that put the mother at risk: eclampsia and retroplacental haematoma.

3°) Complications of pre-eclampsia

Pre-eclampsia can develop rapidly, especially during the third trimester of pregnancy, and in 10% of cases can lead to serious complications that can be life-threatening in the short term for both the mother and her unborn baby. These include eclampsia, which can lead to convulsions or coma, retinal detachment, which can lead to blindness, and cerebral haemorrhage, which is the main cause of maternal death. Liver rupture, kidney failure in the mother, placental abruption causing internal haemorrhage where the placenta was attached. This accident requires an emergency delivery. It should also be noted that a pregnant woman with a BP of 140/90mmHg and proteinuria has a mild form of pre-eclampsia. The presence of proteinuria and an elevated blood pressure of over 140/90 MmHg, combined with visual disturbances, headaches, pain, etc., is a sign of pre-eclampsia. **(Leonid and Anna, September 2016).**

VII- Applicable preventive measures

Since around 2010, it has been possible to screen for pre-eclampsia by measuring various biochemical and obstetric factors. By combining this information, it is possible to assess the risk of a pregnant woman developing pre-eclampsia during her current pregnancy, enabling the doctor to prevent the development of the disease. Screening for pre-eclampsia is carried out in the first trimester, at at least 11 weeks' gestation and less than 14 weeks. It involves a blood test that can be carried out at the same time as screening for trisomy 21 in the 1st trimester of pregnancy. The screening involves measuring the plasma concentration of two biomarkers, the Placental Growth Factor (PlGF) and PAPP-A proteins, and combining these assays with data collected by obstetrician-gynaecologists or midwives: uterine artery Doppler, measurement of the patient's mean arterial pressure, maternal age, smoking habits, geographical origin, BMI, history of hypertension and parity. By combining all these parameters, a predictive risk can be established, as is done for trisomy 21, with a detection rate of up to 96.3%. However, this is a screening test, not a diagnosis. It is therefore important to bear in mind that there is also a rate of false negatives, in other words patients who will not be detected. There is much debate about the value of such screening, given the controversial efficacy of preventive treatment with aspirin. Recent studies have shown that the effectiveness of this treatment depends not only on the dose absorbed, but also on when treatment is started. It is essential to start treatment before 16^{e} weeks of pregnancy in order to achieve a significant reduction in the risk of **(McDonald.SD, 2010).**

You also need :

-Monitor your blood pressure

-Avoid a diet high in salt

- Moderate alcohol consumption

-Giving up smoking

-Adopting a balanced diet

VIII- treatment

Pre-eclampsia is treated in hospital, with close maternal and foetal monitoring. Only the birth of the child can halt the placenta's secretion and the progression of pre-eclampsia towards neurological, hepatic and renal complications. However, complications may arise in the first 48 hours post-partum, and require appropriate monitoring. Before 34 weeks' amenorrhoea, foetal lung maturation using corticosteroids is recommended. In the event of serious complications, emergency foetal extraction may be indicated to save the mother's life. While awaiting a delivery date that is compatible between the life of the child and that of the mother, the latter may be given antihypertensive drugs under medical supervision in hospital. Intravenous magnesium sulphate can limit the onset of eclampsia. In women at risk, taking small doses of aspirin may reduce the risk of pre-eclampsia. Simple treatment with low doses of aspirin, under the direct supervision of your doctor, has been shown to be effective. For this type of treatment to be effective, it must be started before 16 weeks of pregnancy, which is why it is so important to identify at-risk pregnancies early on. Treatment of the crisis eclampsia consists of :

-Clear the airways to avoid asphyxiation;

Administer anti-seizure medication ;

-Carry out an emergency caesarean section as soon as the convulsions have stopped.

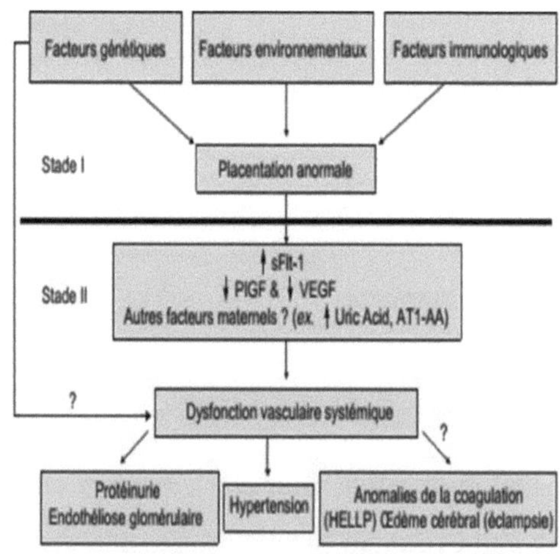

FIG. 2. — Schéma résumant les mécanismes impliqués dans la pathogénie de la pré-éclampsie.

Figure 6: Diagram summarising the mechanism involved in the pathogenesis of pre-eclampsia **(Walker JJ, 2007).**

CHAPTER 2

MATERIALS AND METHODS

I- presentation of the data collection site

We will choose the Protestant hospital in Mbouo, which is located in the western region, Koung-khi department, Poumougne district, at the top of the Bafoussam-Douala No. 3 national road. It is bordered to the north by the Mbouo integrated centre and to the south by the Mbieng health centre. The hospital has several departments, including the laboratory department, where our study will take place, and more specifically the biochemistry and reception departments.

Presentation of the laboratory

Inaugurated on 13 March 2013 by the French Ambassador to Cameroon and Cameroon's Minister of External Relations, under the gaze of the National President of the Evangelical Church of Cameroon and President BIAGNE, the promoter of this work, this architectural jewel uses ten support staff and comprises several departments, namely: biochemistry, serology, parasitology and bacteriology.

-a large waiting room
-a reception room for registering patients, with a staff toilet attached to it

-Three sampling rooms: two for venous sampling and one with a gynaecological table and appropriate equipment for this type of examination.

-The laboratory also has a number of different pieces of equipment for carrying out the examinations specified by the clinician.

Justification for the collection site

We chose this hospital because it is part of one of our application sites, but also because it has a fairly diversified technical platform with a very large number of patients. Given the choice of our topic, it would be beneficial for everyone to conduct our study in this institute.

II- sampling method

The sampling method we used was a non-probability method: all pregnant women who came to the Mbouo Protestant Hospital for a consultation and who agreed to take part in our study were included in our sample.

Sampling technique

The sample size was calculated using an estimated prevalence of pre-eclampsia in Black Africa of between 2.8 and 6.1%. Using the formula of **LORENTZ,**

$$N=Z^2P\ (1-P)/d^2$$

N=sample size

Z=confidence level: for a confidence level of 95%, Z=1.96 P=prevalence of the health problem in the population

d = tolerated margin of error. For a Z=95%, d=0.05

With this prevalence, our sample size will be 87.

Type and duration of study

Our aim was to carry out a cross-sectional and analytical study in two stages: a survey phase and a second phase involving the collection of specimens (blood and urine) suitable for our study. The collection period ran from July 2016 to September 2016.

Source population: our source population consisted of all people who came to the Mbouo Protestant Hospital for consultations.

Target population: all pregnant women attending the Mbouo Protestant Hospital.

Study population: all pregnant women attending the Mbouo Protestant Hospital who agreed to take part in our study.

Non-inclusion criteria

- All female patients who are not pregnant

-male patients

Inclusion criteria

-being a patient pregnant woman

-visit our collection site during our study period

-agree to take part in our study.

III- Ethical consideration of research

In order to carry out our study, we obtained authorisation from the regional public health delegate by means of a letter written to him and signed by the director of the private health staff training complex in Mbouo, plus a copy of our protocol. After this, we went to the management of the Mbouo Protestant Hospital to request authorisation from the director, who allowed us to carry out our study in his institution. All the patients in our study were given a confidential identification code. This same code was applied to the sample received in the laboratory. These patients were told about the purpose of the research, its interest and the importance of their participation in the study. In the light of all this, they gave If they were in favour, they filled in the questionnaire provided for this purpose. effect. By signing it, they acknowledged that they had given their approval for their participation in the study.

IV- work methodology Pre-analytical phase

This phase consisted of welcoming and registering the patient, giving her an identification code, providing her with the necessary conditions for carrying out the test, labelling the tubes and boxes needed to collect the specimen, explaining the purpose of the test and taking the sample.

Analytical phase

Here, we used uric acid measurement, blood pressure monitoring and protein measurement in the urine of these women as biological markers, the elevation of which indicated a risk of pre-eclampsia. This phase consisted of collecting the specimen required for the test (the whole blood would be centrifuged at 3,000 rpm and the serum obtained would be used to measure uric acid using a spectrophotometer). The urine obtained will not be centrifuged, but analysed directly. The women's blood pressure will be recorded in their diaries immediately after the consultation.

Procedure for the determination of uric acid.

The test we are going to use here is **INMESCO Gmbh-wiedtalstr.**

manufactured by **Neustadt/wied-Germany.**

Specimen collection and preparation: non-haemolyzed serum, plasma collected on EDTA or heparin

Interference: high levels of bilirubin and/or ascorbic acid interfere negatively with the assay. Results may be overestimated in cases of high lipemia or haemolysis of the specimen. In patients who have been treated with vitamin c, interference due to ascorbic acid may occur. ascorbic acid can be reduced by leaving the specimen at room temperature for 2 hours before carrying out the assay.

Principle of the test: Uric acid is oxidised by uricase into allantoin and hydrogen peroxide under the influence of pod4-amino-phenazone and 2,4dichlorophenol sulphonate. A red precipitate is formed, which is quinonemine. The intensity of the coloration is proportional to the concentration of uric acid and will be read at a wavelength of 520 nm. **Procedure:** bring the reagents and/or specimen to room temperature.

Measure in well-identified test tubes	White	Stallion	dosage
Reagent from work	1ml	1ml	1ml
Specimen(Rq1)			20μl
Stallion		20μl	
Water demineralised	20μl		
Mix and leave to rest for 5 minutes at 25°c Read the absorbance at 520 nm (490-530) against the reagent white Colour is stable for 30 minutes			

Calculation: the result will be determined using the following formula

Serum and plasma: result =A sample*concentration of standard/A standard

C=60 mg/l=6 mg/dl=357μmol/l

Normal value: 2.3-6.1 mg/l or 137 to 363μmol/l

To make the combi 10, the kit box contains strips containing 10 parameters, and the part we are concerned with will be that corresponding to proteins and glucose. This strip will be dipped into the urine and the colour change will be observed and compared with the values written on the reagent box. (See attached technical data sheet) We used **CYBOW** urine strips to measure proteinuria. According to this reagent, normal urine contains protein and the normal value is <20mg/dl.Above this value, there is already an indication of pathology.

Post-analysis phase

In this case, it was the results that pointed to a risk for our pathology, which was being studied. All patients at risk were referred to the doctor for treatment. Those who were not at risk were given prophylactic measures by us to avoid this pathology.

Data processing

The data collected was recorded in a notebook and then entered using Microsoft Office 2010 Word and Excel software. Analysis

Statistical analysis was carried out using SPSS software toassess the extent to which the population is affected by the disease.

-Declaration of variables

BMI=body mass **index**. According to the WHO, this is the abnormal or excessive accumulation of body fat that represents a health risk and is calculated by the formula: BMI=P/T² (with p=weight in kilograms and t=height in metres). According to the WHO, the normal value for pregnant women is between 18 and 25. Below 18, we talk about a state of cachexia; between 25 and 30, we talk about overweight and above 30, we talk about obesity **(WHO June 2012).**

Proteinuria: normal value <20mg/dl according to the **CYBOW** reagent **Blood pressure**: normal value in pregnant women :

PAS<140mmhg and PAD< to 90 mmHg (**CLAIRE MOUNIER, vascular medicine and hypertension; 2009**)

Uric acid: according to the **INMESCO** GmbH-wiedtalstr reagent we used, the normal value is between 2.3-6.1 mg/dl.

Odd Ratio(OR) =Frequency of exposed/1-frequency exposed/Frequency unexposed/1-frequency unexposed

CHAPTER 3

RESULTS AND INTERPRETATION

Our survey enabled us to collect 86 pregnant women and to characterise them as follows:

I- socio-demographic characteristics

❖ **place of residence**

Figure 17 shows that the Mbieng district was the most represented with a percentage of 29%, while the Baleng district was the least represented with only 3%. We can therefore say that the majority of our study population came from the rural area, i.e. 93% of our respondents, and only 13% came from the urban area.

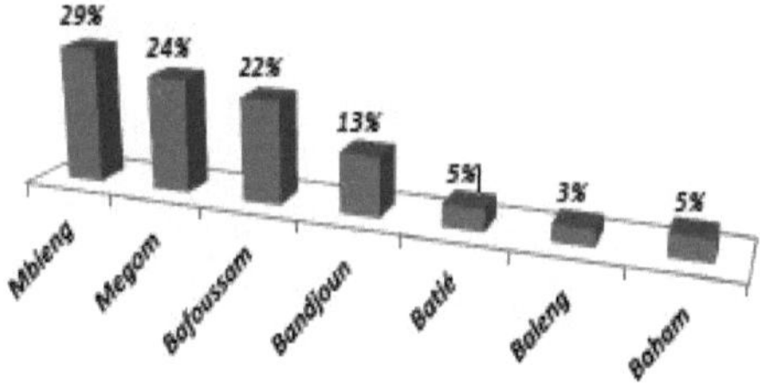

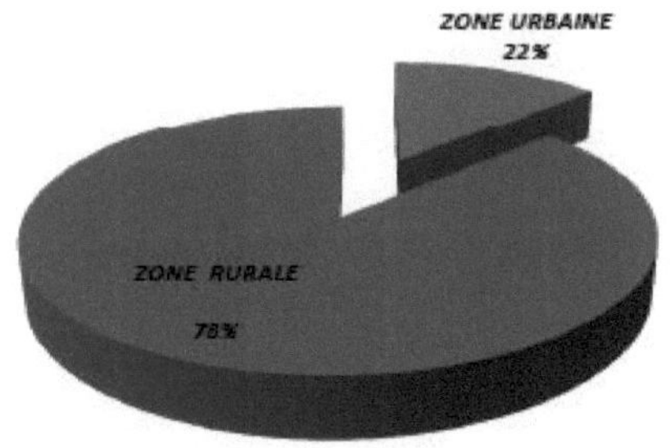

Figure 17: Breakdown of women by place of residence

❖ **profession**

Most of our respondents during our collection period were housewives, representing 61% of our study population. Next came female teachers (11%), followed by female students (only 2%).

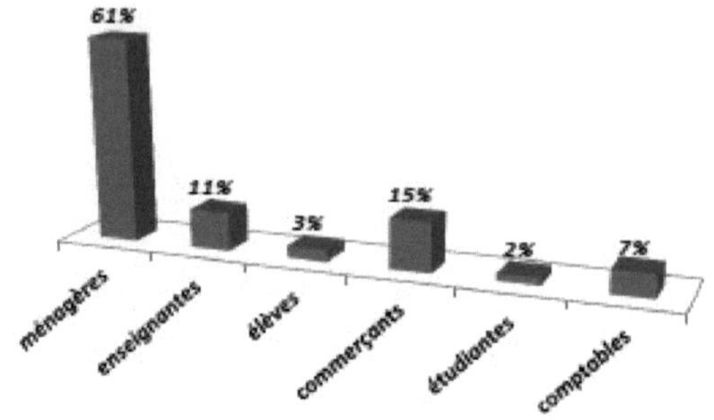

Figure 8: Breakdown of women by profession

❖ **age**

The most represented age group was between 22 and 26. The mean age was 28.28 (ranging from 17 to 43 years), with a standard deviation of 5.485.

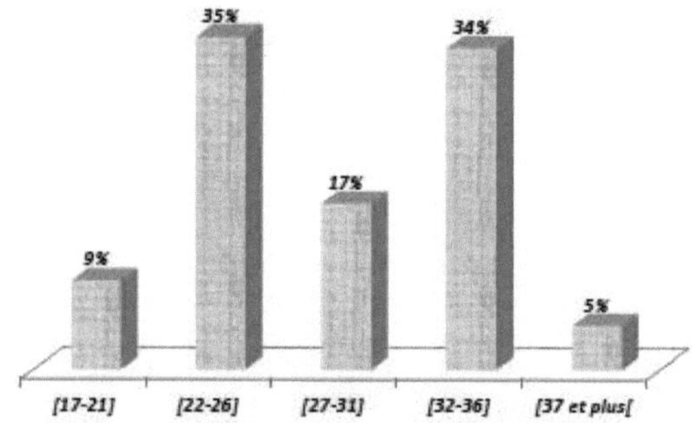

Figure 9: Breakdown of respondents by age group

❖ **knowledge about preeclampsia :**

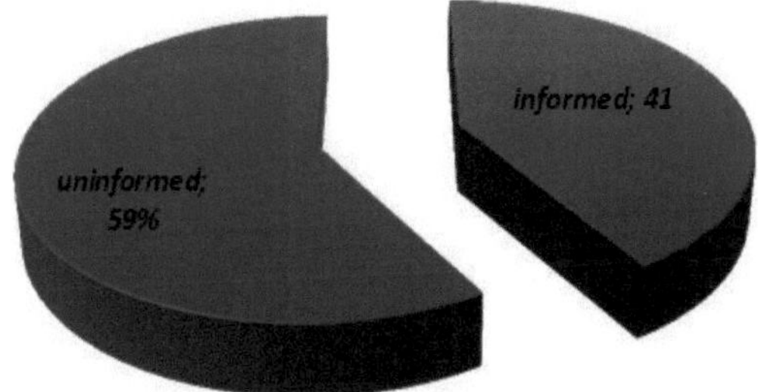

Figure 10: Distribution of women according to their knowledge of pre-eclampsia

❖ **Marital status**

Most of these women were married, representing 51% of our study population. Followed by single women (36%) and engaged women (14%).

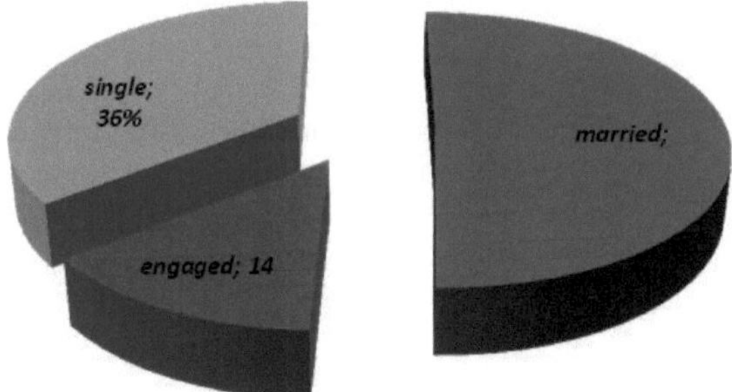

Figure11 : distribution of respondents in according to of their marital status

II- obstetrical history

Figure 11 shows the history of pregnancy hypertension, abortion, death in utero, caesarean section and prematurity. We can see that a history of arterial hypertension was the most frequent with a percentage of 28% of the total population; followed by a history of caesarean section with 6%. A history of death in utero and caesarean section were not overly represented with a frequency of 1% each.

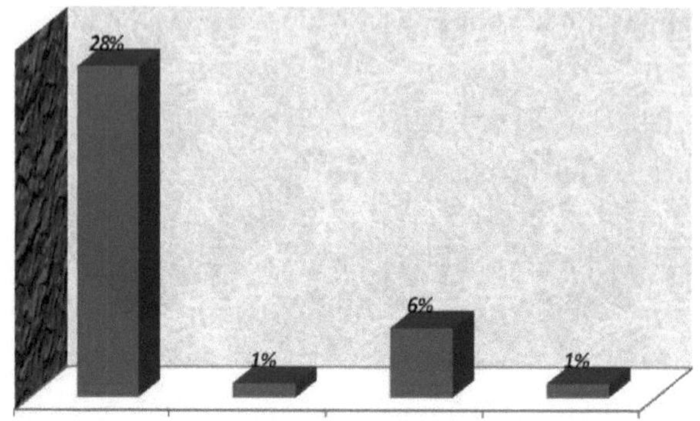

Htamort in utero caesarean sections premature

Figure 12:Distribution of respondents in according to of obstetrical history

A-Risk factors

-BMI

Table 1: Distribution of respondents according to their BMI

type of imc					
workforce		Percentage	Valid percentage	Cumulative percentage	Frequencies
normal	43	50	50	50	50%
overweight	30	34,9	34,9	84,9	35%
obese	13	15,1	15,1	100	15%
Total	86	100	100		100%

Calculating the body mass index of each of these pregnant women enabled us to find the number of overweight, obese and low-body mass women. The table shows that 30 of the 86 women were overweight, representing 35% of our study population. 13 of these women were obese, representing 15% of our sample, and 43 were of normal weight, representing 50% of our study population. Almost half of our respondents (50%) had a normal BMI.

Table2:distribution of BMI in according to of brackets age

workfor ce				type of imc			
			Normal		overweight		obese
		N	%	N	%	N	%
	17-21	4	9%	4	13%	0	0%
	22-26	15	35%	9	30%	6	46%
Tranche age	27-31	8	19%	7	23%	0	0%
	32-36	14	33%	8	27%	7	54%
	37 and more	2	5%	2	7%	0	0%
total		43	100%	30	100%	13	100%

The table shows that the age group most affected by overweight is between 22 and 26 and the age group most affected by obesity is between 32 and 36. We can therefore say that age does not have a significant influence on BMI (Chi-square read=15.51>Calculated Chi-square 8.19 ,ddl=8).

B-Other risk factors

Most of the pregnant women in our sample were having their first pregnancy, representing 22% of the women in our sample. This was followed by women with twin pregnancies, who accounted for 12% of our sample. Pregnant women with diabetes accounted for only 07%. of our study population, and women with oedema represented 10% of our study population.

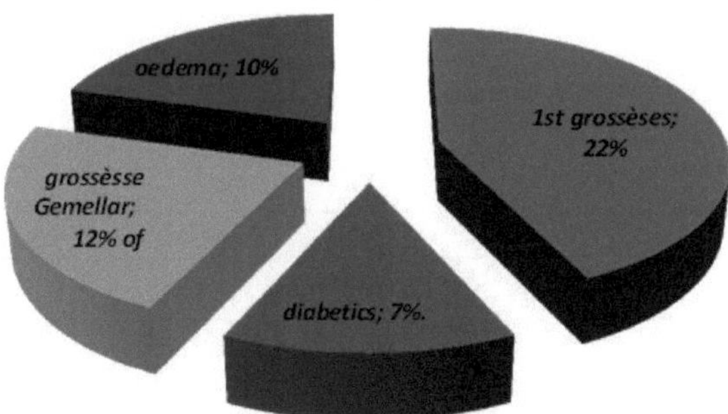

Figure 13: Distribution of respondents according to risk factors for pre-eclampsia

C-E assessment of the diagnosis

-high blood pressure

The distribution of blood pressure as a function of SBP and DBP enabled us to characterise the type of blood pressure in these pregnant women. The figure opposite shows the blood pressure characteristics of these pregnant women. It shows that 91% had normal blood pressure, 5% had mild hypertension and 3% had moderate hypertension. It should also be noted that 1% of these women had hypotension.

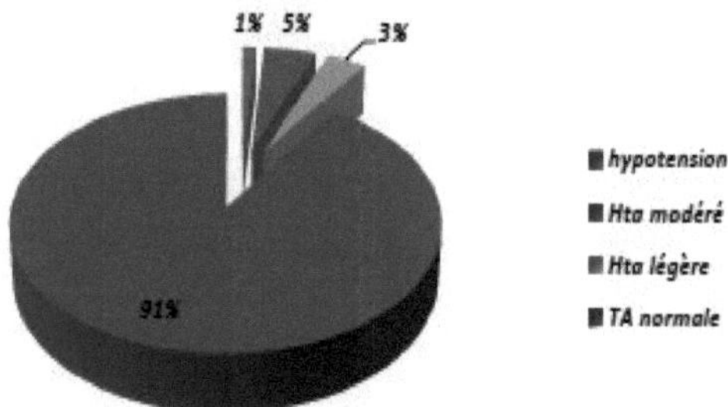

Figure 14: Distribution according to blood pressure characteristics in these pregnant women

Table 3: Breakdown by uric acid level

uric acid					
Frequency		Percentage	Valid percentage	Cumulative percentage	Frequency
High	25	29,1	29,1	29,1	29%
Low	6	7,0	7,0	36,0	7%
Normal	55	64,0	64,0	100,0	64%
Total	86	100,0	100,0		100%

Measuring uric acid levels in these pregnant women enabled us to classify their uric acid levels into several stages. Those with low uric acid levels represented 9% of our sample. Next came 31% with high uric acid levels and 59% with normal uric acid levels.

Table 4: Proteinuria distribution

Frequency		Percentage	Percentage valid	Cumulative percentage	Frequency
100	6	7,0	7,0	7,0	7%
30	4	4,7	4,7	11,6	5%
Negati f	73	84,9	84,9	96,5	85%
Trace	3	3,5	3,5	100,0	3%
Total	86	100,0	100,0		100%

From this figure, we can see that 12% of our respondents had high proteinuria, followed by 3% who had mild proteinuria. We can also say that 85% had normal proteinuria.

Uric acid + hta

Of these 86 pregnant women, we recorded 64% who had a normal uric acid + normal BP combination, i.e. 55 respondents. 7% had a low uric acid level and normal BP, i.e. 6 respondents. 3 had high uric acid and mild hypertension (3.4%), 4 had high uric acid and moderate hypertension (4, 65%) and 17 had high uric acid and normal blood pressure (19%), making a total of 29% of our study population. We can also say that uric acid has a significant influence on BP (P=0.001<0.05) ddl=6

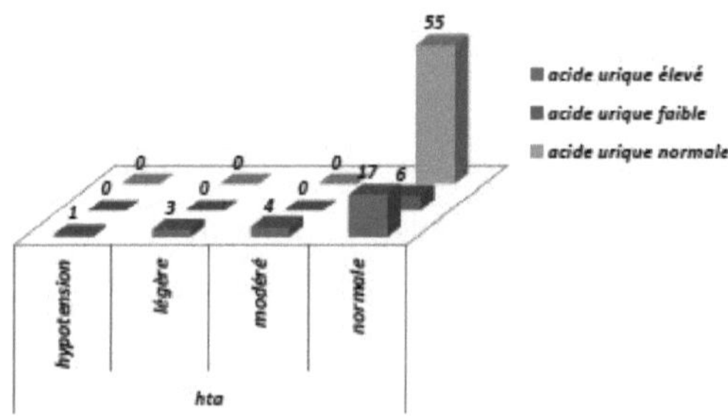

Figure 15: Representation of the association between uric acid and blood pressure in our respondents

-hta and proteinuria

The figure below shows the association of proteinuria and blood pressure in our respondents. We can say that one woman out of 86 presented an association of normal proteinuria + hypotension which represented 1.16% of our respondents.71 presented an association of normal proteinuria and normal blood pressure which represented 82.55% of our respondents.3 women out of 86 had mild proteinuria and normal blood pressure, representing 3.48% of our respondents.Elevated proteinuria and mild blood pressure was observed in 2 of our respondents, representing 2.32%.4 respondents out of 86 had an association of elevated proteinuria and normal blood pressure, representing 4.65% of our respondents.4 others had elevated proteinuria and normal blood pressure. Normal or4,65%of our sample.the proteinuria significantly influence BP with a P=0.001<0.05.ddl=6

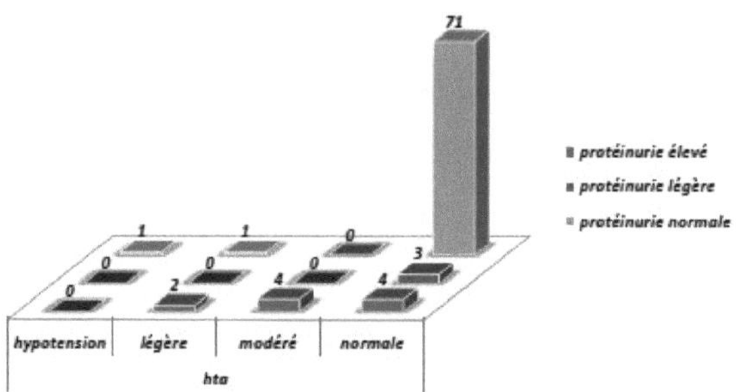

Figure 16: Representation of the association between proteinuria and blood pressure in our respondents

-Uric acid and proteinuria

The figure below shows that 6 out of 86 women had low uric acid levels and normal proteinuria, i.e. 6.97% of our respondents. 8 out of 86 had high uric acid levels and high proteinuria, i.e. 9.30%. There were also 16 respondents with high uric acid levels and normal proteinuria, i.e. 18.6%. 51 out of 86 of our respondents had normal uric acid levels and normal proteinuria, i.e. 59.30% of our sample. Uric acid had no significant influence on proteinuria (G.beucher, 2010)(P=0.06>0.05 ddl=4).

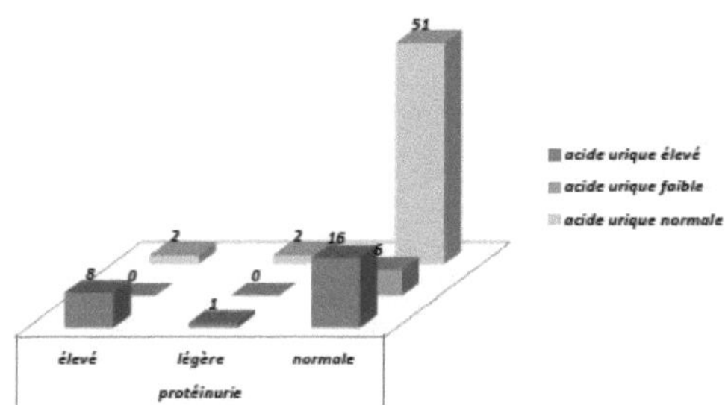

Figure 17: representation of the uric acid proteinuria association in our respondents

Table 5: Cross-tabulation of uric acid*Hta*Proteinuria in our respondents

Workforce							
			Hta				
Proteinuria			hypotension	slight	moderate	normal	Total
High	uric acid	high		2	4	2	8
		normal		0	0	2	2
	Total			2	4	4	10
Slight	uric acid	high				1	1
		normal				2	2
	Total					3	3
Normal	uric acid	high	1	1		14	16
		low	0	0		6	6
		normal	0	0		51	51
	Total		1	1		71	73
Total	uric acid	high	1	3	4	17	25
		low	0	0	0	6	6
		normal	0	0	0	55	55
	Total		1	3	4	78	86

From this table, we can see that six of our 86 respondents had an association of our three markers under study (HT, hyperuricemia, proteinuria), representing 6.97% of our study population.

CHAPTER 4

DISCUSSION

The aim of our study was to contribute to the prevention of pre-eclampsia in pregnant women.

-Breakdown of respondents by profession and place of residence

The most represented profession in our study was that of housewife, with a percentage of 61%, followed by shopkeepers (15%). Most of these women lived in rural areas, i.e. 78% of our respondents, compared with the work of **Mamie Ngunga Nkondi, who in 2005** worked in the DRC on pregnant women who were all civil servants in urban areas.

-Breakdown by age.

The age of the patients varied between 17 and 40 years (which gives us an average of 28.5%). The most represented age group was between 22 and 26 years, which is approximately equal to that found by (Auger .N, 2015) who worked in genesis and found an average age of 29.5 (extreme 20 and 39 years).

-Breakdown by marital status

During our study, the most common marital status was married (51%). 14% were engaged women who had not yet registered. 36% were unmarried. This is similar to the work **of Daniel Vaiman in 2014**, who worked on all pregnant women from the twentieth week of amenorrhoea without distinction of marital status.

-Breakdown by risk factor

One of the aims of this study was to assess the factors favouring the onset of pre-eclampsia. The most significant risk factors for developing pre-eclampsia were obesity and overweight before pregnancy (OR respectively equal to 0.17

and 0.51), which is lower than that found by **Bodnar L., Ness R in 2008 in Angola** (OR=2.61 and 2.50).the age group most affected by these factors was between [32-36y] and [22-26y] which is approximately equal to that found by **Van Vugt J.M** in **2007** in New Zealand [30- 35y] and [23-27y].this obesity and overweight may be related to an unbalanced diet in these pregnant women, the purchasing power of our respondents, ignorance and the culture of availability. More recently, **Thadhani et al** in **2009** found a relative risk of developing pre-eclampsia of two when the pre-pregnancy BMI was greater than 25 and a relative risk of 2.6 when it was greater than 30. Several hypotheses have been put forward to explain this: some postulate that hypertension occurs during pregnancy in the obese patient due to an increase in cardiac output, while others (and this is the hypothesis most widely accepted) believe that hyperlipidaemia favours the production of peroxides, leading to an alteration in the endothelium and vasoconstriction. **Dugoff L., Hobbins J 2008. L TOUZART** in his 2008 study found a risk of developing pre-eclampsia in women with at least one personal history of pre-eclampsia (OR=8.12).The first pregnancy was observed between the ages of 22 and 26, which is lower than the work of **Levine R.J. in 2008 in Cape Verde**, who observed a first pregnancy between the ages of 27 and 30. This may be due to the fact that education does not or negligence. There have been two cases of diabetes in which The age was between 22 and 26, which was not too significant because their blood glucose levels had not been checked afterwards due to our short collection period.In our sample, we also found a link between preeclampsia and the existence of at least one family history of chronic arterial hypertension and caesarean section in a female relative, with an OR of 0.31 which is lower than that found by **Ness R.B., Markovic N** in 2008 (OR=2.63). This element has been much less described in the literature, although a few publications corroborate this finding. For example, a recent study by **Ness R.B., Markovic N** in 2008 reported a strong association between the risk of cardiovascular disease in a woman's first-degree relatives and her own risk of pre-eclampsia. According to this analysis, having two or more family members with cardiovascular disease risk factors (hypertension, diabetes, stroke) versus having no family members at all increases the probability of developing pre-eclampsia (OR: 1.9).The association of hyperuricemia + arterial hypertension + proteinuria observed in 6.97% of our sample represented an OR of 0.05, which is approximately equal to that found by **PEIRIS H** in 2007 (OR=0.059). The range in which this association of three factors was high was between [24-40], higher than that found by **NGUNGA NKONDI** in 2005 in the DRC, where the association of the three markers was observed in the under-20s. This may be due to the type of food consumed by pregnant women, who, during pregnancy, love protein-rich foods such as pork (animal offal), resulting in hyperuricaemia, which may subsequently lead to arterial hypertension. With a view to improving the predictivity of these clinical factors, researchers such as **Lambert-Messerlian G., Silver H., Petraglia F., Luisi S., Pezzani I. and Canick J**. conducted a prospective study from 2000 to 2010 in **Boston, USA,** on biological markers in the first trimester of pregnancy in order to determine whether their association would increase the prediction of this pathology. These markers are βhCG, inhibin A, pregnancy-associated plasma protein A (PAPP-A), C-reactive protein (CRP) and placental growth factor.and markers such as PIGF: Placental Growth Factor sFlt-1: fms-like tyrosine kinase 1 - (Soluble fraction of the VEGF membrane receptor (VEGFR), PAPP-A: Pregnancy Associated Plasma Protein A - (Type A placental plasma protein) were proven by Dr **François TOSETTI on 18 March 2014** to be true markers of EP in the 1er trimester of pregnancy.

CONCLUSION

This study evaluated the biological diagnosis and risk factors for pre-eclampsia, which is caused by the placenta. Once the placenta has been expelled, the mother's condition is rapidly resolved, although she will continue to be monitored for some time to ensure that the hypertension has disappeared. In the event of a new pregnancy, the chances of recurrence are minimal, if not non-existent. However, if a woman has suffered from pre-eclampsia during a previous pregnancy, subsequent pregnancies will continue to be closely monitored, to avoid taking any further risks.

RECOMMENDATION

In order to reduce maternal and foetal morbidity and mortality linked to this pathology, we recommend the following:

-At the Mbouo Protestant Hospital:

Promote multidisciplinary management (obstetricians, paediatricians, intensive care specialists) of severe cases of pre-eclampsia

-Draw up a protocol for managing cases of gestational hypertension and display it or make it available in the maternity department in order to standardise the action to be taken according to the clinical picture.

To make available and promote the use of magnesium sulphate in cases of eclampsia or severe pre-eclampsia with signs of threatened eclampsia.

-Provide the maternity unit with sufficient, competent and motivated staff.

-Ministry of Public Health :

Provide training for all those responsible for carrying out prenatal consultations to improve their quality, so that they can detect mothers-to-be who are at risk, in order to detect cases at an early stage. to refer them as quickly as possible to a health facility capable of treating them properly.

-to provide hospitals with kits for measuring PAPP-A, VEGFR, PIGF and SFLT-1 in order to diagnose this pathology earlier (in the first trimester of pregnancy) for proper management.

REFERENCE

1. Abalos E, C. C. (2009). Short-term outcome of patients with pre-eclampsia. london: ANN epidemiol.

2. Agnès Ditisheim, A. P.-B. (2014, April). Retrieved September 12, 2016, from www.hug-ge.ch/endocrinologie-diabetologie-hypertension-: http://contrepoids.

3. Auger .N, F. W. (2015). Association between preeclampsia and congenital heart defects. PARIS: JAMA.

4. Bainbridge S, S. (2013). Global and regional estimates of pre-eclampsia and eclampsia. Eur J obset , 1-7.

5. BENIRSCHKE K, K. P. (2008). Nonvillous parts and trophoblast. Newyork, USA: SpringerVerlag.

6. Bodnar.l, N. (2008) . The risk of preeclampsia rises with increasing prepregnancy body mass index. london, england: Ann epidemiol.

7. Daniel Vaiman, d. d. (2014). pre-eclampsia. (INSERM, Ed.) PARIS, COCHIN, FRANCE.

8. ducarne, G. e. (2009). Revisiting the epidemiological standard of preeclampsia. london: adventure works press.

9. G.beucher, T. (2010). Formalised expert recommendations. copenhagen: ann Fr annesth.

10. J.Clin, M. C. (2005). Hyperuricemia and xanthine oxidase in preeclampsia (D. Junca) denmark: Ann gynecol.

11. Kaiman, D. (2014). Pre-eclampsia. paris, france: Adventure work press.

12. Kajantie E, E. J. (2009). "Pre-eclampsia is associated with increased risk of stroke in the adult offspring. the Helsinki birth cohort study.

13. Lambert-Messerlian G., S. H. (2000 to 2010). Second-trimester levels of maternal serum hCG and inhibin A as predictors of preeclampsia in the third trimester of pregnancy. Boston, USA: Soc gynécol invest.

14. Levine R.J., T. R. (2008). Urinary placental growth factor and risk of preeclampsia. JAMA.

15. MAYNARD SE, M. J. (2006). Excess placental soluble fms-like tyrosine kinase 1 (sFlt1) may contribute to endothelial dysfunction, hypertension, and proteinuria in preeclampsi. J CLIN INVEST.

16. McDonald.SD, H. E. (2010). Circulating angiogenic factors and the risk of preeclampsia. N Engl J Med.

17. MOUNIER, C. (2009). vascular medicine and hypertension. PARIS.

18. Ness R.B, M. N. (2008). amily history of hypertension, heart disease, and stroke among women who develop hypertension in pregnancy (Vol. III). obstet gynécol.

19. NKONDI, M. N. (2005). Maternal and fetal prognosis during severe pre-eclampsia. Retrieved July 2016, from www.mémoireonlone.com.

20. Schaffer N, D. J. (2008). URIC acid clearance in normal pregnancy and preeclampsia. geneva: soc Gynecl invest.

21. Thadani R, S,.(2009). Risk of hypertensive disorders of pregnancy. london: obset gynecol.

22. TOSSETTI, F. (2014). PARIS: CPDN.

23. Van vugt, J. (2007). levated CRP levels during first trimester of pregnancy are indicative of preeclampsia and intrauterine growth restriction. poland: J-reprod Immunol.

24. www.medhyg.ch/formation/article.php3?sid=33881. (s.d.).

25. www.socnephrologie.org/PDF/epart/industries/gambro-pdf.(2011, JANUARY). Retrieved on APRIL 2016, from www.socnephrologie.org: http://www.socnephrologie.org

APPENDIX

TIMETABLES AND BUDGET ON

Timeline :

MONTHS	ELABORATION OF THE PROTOCOLE	DATA COLLECTION	DATA PROCESSING	REDACTION OF MEMORY	SOUTENANCE
APRIL 2016	□				
AUGUST 2016		□			
OCTOBER 2016			□		
JANUARY 2016				□	
MAY 2016					□

Estimated budget for the work

Uric acid reagent	20000fcfa
1l alcohol	1000fcfa
Dry cotton	500fcfa
100 dry tubes	5000fcfa
Combi 2	10000fcfa
Yellow and blue tips	9000fcfa
A ream of	2500fcfa
Unforeseen	10000fcfa
1 pack of gang	2500fcfa
1 pack of syringes	4500fcfa
Urine pots(100)	10000fcfa
Total	75000fcfa

Consent form

I, the undersigned (Code)

I hereby certify that I have understood the importance of this study and that I have had the opportunity to ask any questions I may have had.

I understand the objectives, risks and potential benefits of taking part in this study.

I agree that the biological product (blood) removed from me may be used in the study.

I accept that the anonymous data recorded during this survey may be processed electronically.

I have noted that I can access this data at any time by contacting the laboratory where the study is being carried out.

I freely agree to take part in this study

I agree that any doctor or scientist involved in the conduct of this research, as well as representatives of the health authorities, may have access to the information in the strictest confidence.

Done at le

The investigator:Participant's signature

KAMGA BRICE CABREL

Survey form

Anonymity..........................

Last name ....

First name...................................

Age...

Number of week of amenorrhoea.

1- have you ever heard of pre-eclampsia?yes n

2- have you ever had a congenital malformation? Yes no

3- during your pregnancy, did you experience any unusual or persistent headaches? yes No

4- do you have swollen feet, hands or ankles (oedema)? no

5- Do you have any visual problems such as blurred vision, flying flies or flashes of light? YesNo

6- are you feeling generally unwell? Yes No

7- do you have pain in the upper abdomen or under the rib on the right? Yes

8- are you pregnant for the first time? yes no

If not you are at the date................

9- has anyone in your family ever had a malformed or stillborn child? yes no

10- is a member of your family already diedafter giving birth?yes no

11- have you ever had a voluntary or involuntary termination of pregnancy? Yes No

Results :

BP normal value

Proteinuria: positive negative

Uric acid Normal value

Signature

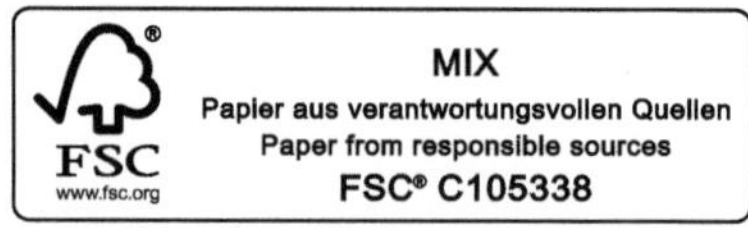

Printed by Books on Demand GmbH, Norderstedt / Germany